Table of Contents

Low Tyramine Recipes

1. Grilled Chicken Salad

Ingredients:

- 4 oz grilled chicken breast, sliced
- 2 cups mixed salad greens
- 1/2 cup cherry tomatoes, halved
- 1/4 cucumber, sliced
- 1/4 avocado, diced
- 2 tablespoons balsamic vinaigrette dressing (low-tyramine)

Instructions:

- Arrange mixed salad greens on a plate or in a bowl.
- Top with sliced grilled chicken breast, cherry tomatoes, cucumber, and diced avocado.
- Drizzle with balsamic vinaigrette dressing.
- Serve immediately, with whole-grain bread or crackers on the side if desired.

2. Baked Salmon with Quinoa and Steamed Vegetables

Ingredients:

- 4 oz salmon fillet
- 1/2 cup quinoa, rinsed
- 1 cup low-sodium vegetable broth
- 1 cup mixed vegetables (such as broccoli, carrots, and bell peppers)
- 1 tablespoon olive oil
- Salt and pepper to taste

Instructions:

- Preheat oven to 375°F (190°C). Place salmon fillet on a baking sheet lined with parchment paper. Season with salt, pepper, and a drizzle of olive oil.
- In a saucepan, bring vegetable broth to a boil. Stir in quinoa, reduce heat to low, cover, and simmer for 15 minutes or until quinoa is cooked and liquid is absorbed.
- While the quinoa is cooking, steam mixed vegetables until tender-crisp, about 5-7 minutes.
- Serve baked salmon alongside cooked quinoa and steamed vegetables.

3. Spinach and Feta Omelette

Ingredients:

- 2 large eggs

- 1/4 cup fresh spinach, chopped
- 2 tablespoons crumbled feta cheese
- 1 tablespoon diced tomatoes
- Salt and pepper to taste
- 1 teaspoon olive oil

Instructions:

- In a bowl, whisk together eggs, chopped spinach, and crumbled feta cheese. Season with salt and pepper.
- Heat olive oil in a non-stick skillet over medium heat. Pour egg mixture into the skillet.
- Cook the omelette for 2-3 minutes, or until the edges start to set. Sprinkle diced tomatoes over one half of the omelette.
- Carefully fold the other half of the omelette over the tomatoes. Cook for another 1-2 minutes, or until the omelette is cooked through.
- Slide the omelette onto a plate and serve hot.

4. Turkey and Avocado Wrap

Ingredients:

- 1 whole grain or low-tyramine wrap
- 3 oz sliced turkey breast
- 1/4 avocado, sliced
- 1/4 cup shredded lettuce
- 1 tablespoon hummus
- 1 teaspoon Dijon mustard

Instructions:

- Lay the wrap flat on a clean surface. Spread hummus evenly over the center of the wrap.
- Layer sliced turkey breast, avocado slices, and shredded lettuce on top of the hummus.
- Drizzle Dijon mustard over the filling ingredients.
- Fold the sides of the wrap towards the center, then roll it up tightly.
- Slice the wrap in half diagonally and serve with carrot sticks or cucumber slices on the side.

5. Vegetable Stir-Fry with Tofu

Ingredients:

- 1/2 block firm tofu, drained and cubed
- 2 cups mixed vegetables (such as bell peppers, snap peas, carrots, and broccoli)
- 2 tablespoons low-sodium soy sauce
- 1 tablespoon hoisin sauce
- 1 teaspoon sesame oil
- 1 clove garlic, minced
- Cooked brown rice or quinoa, for serving

Instructions:

- Heat sesame oil in a large skillet or wok over medium heat. Add minced garlic and cubed tofu to the skillet.
- Stir-fry tofu until golden brown on all sides, about 5-7 minutes. Remove tofu from the skillet and set aside.
- In the same skillet, add mixed vegetables and stir-fry until crisp-tender, about 3-4 minutes.
- Return tofu to the skillet with the vegetables. Add soy sauce and hoisin sauce, stirring to coat evenly.
- Cook for an additional 1-2 minutes, until the sauce is heated through.
- Serve the vegetable stir-fry over cooked brown rice or quinoa.

6. Veggie Sticks with Hummus

Ingredients:

- Carrot sticks
- Cucumber sticks
- Bell pepper strips
- Cherry tomatoes
- 1/4 cup homemade or store-bought hummus

Instructions:

- Wash and prepare the vegetables by cutting them into sticks or strips.
- Arrange the veggie sticks on a plate alongside cherry tomatoes.
- Serve with a side of hummus for dipping.

7. Lemon Herb Grilled Chicken

Ingredients:

- 2 boneless, skinless chicken breasts
- 2 tablespoons olive oil
- 2 tablespoons lemon juice
- 2 cloves garlic, minced
- 1 teaspoon dried oregano
- 1 teaspoon dried thyme
- Salt and pepper to taste

Instructions:

- In a small bowl, whisk together olive oil, lemon juice, minced garlic, dried oregano, dried thyme, salt, and pepper to create the marinade.
- Place chicken breasts in a shallow dish and pour the marinade over them, turning to coat evenly. Cover and refrigerate for at least 30 minutes, or up to 4 hours.
- Preheat grill to medium-high heat. Remove chicken from marinade and discard excess marinade.
- Grill chicken breasts for 6-8 minutes per side, or until cooked through and no longer pink in the center.
- Remove from grill and let rest for a few minutes before serving. Slice and serve with your choice of side dishes.

8. Berry Parfait

Ingredients:

- 1/2 cup plain Greek yogurt (low-tyramine)
- 1/4 cup granola (low-tyramine)
- 1/2 cup mixed berries (such as strawberries, blueberries, raspberries)
- 1 tablespoon honey or maple syrup (optional)

Instructions:

- In a glass or bowl, layer Greek yogurt, granola, and mixed berries.
- Repeat layers until ingredients are used up, ending with a layer of berries on top.
- Drizzle honey or maple syrup over the top for added sweetness, if desired.
- Serve immediately as a nutritious and satisfying dessert option.

9. Veggie Breakfast Scramble

Ingredients:

- 2 large eggs
- 1/4 cup diced bell peppers (any color)
- 1/4 cup diced onions
- 1/4 cup sliced mushrooms

- 1/4 cup diced tomatoes
- Salt and pepper to taste
- 1 teaspoon olive oil

Instructions:

- Heat olive oil in a non-stick skillet over medium heat.
- Add diced onions, bell peppers, and mushrooms to the skillet. Sauté until vegetables are tender, about 5 minutes.
- In a bowl, whisk together eggs with diced tomatoes, salt, and pepper.
- Pour the egg mixture into the skillet with the sautéed vegetables. Cook, stirring occasionally, until eggs are set and scrambled.
- Serve hot with whole-grain toast or a side of fresh fruit.

10. Quinoa Salad with Chickpeas and Feta

Ingredients:

- 1 cup cooked quinoa, cooled
- 1/2 cup canned chickpeas, drained and rinsed
- 1/4 cup crumbled feta cheese
- 1/4 cup diced cucumber
- 1/4 cup halved cherry tomatoes
- 2 tablespoons chopped fresh parsley
- 1 tablespoon extra virgin olive oil
- 1 tablespoon lemon juice
- Salt and pepper to taste

Instructions:

- In a large bowl, combine cooked quinoa, chickpeas, crumbled feta cheese, diced cucumber, cherry tomatoes, and chopped fresh parsley.
- Drizzle extra virgin olive oil and lemon juice over the salad. Season with salt and pepper to taste.
- Toss the salad gently to combine all the ingredients.
- Serve chilled or at room temperature as a refreshing and nutritious lunch option.

11.   Lentil Vegetable Soup

Ingredients:

- 1 cup dried lentils, rinsed
- 4 cups low-sodium vegetable broth
- 1 onion, diced
- 2 carrots, diced
- 2 celery stalks, diced
- 2 cloves garlic, minced
- 1 teaspoon dried thyme
- 1 teaspoon dried oregano
- Salt and pepper to taste
- 2 tablespoons chopped fresh parsley (for garnish)

Instructions:

- In a large pot, combine dried lentils, vegetable broth, diced onion, carrots, celery, minced garlic, dried thyme, and dried oregano.
- Bring the soup to a boil, then reduce heat to low and simmer for 20-25 minutes, or until lentils and vegetables are tender.
- Season the soup with salt and pepper to taste.
- Ladle the soup into bowls and garnish with chopped fresh parsley before serving. Serve hot with crusty whole-grain bread on the side.

12. Cottage Cheese and Fruit Bowl

Ingredients:

- 1/2 cup low-fat cottage cheese
- 1/2 cup sliced fresh fruit (such as pineapple, strawberries, or peaches)
- 1 tablespoon chopped nuts (such as almonds or walnuts) (optional)
- 1 teaspoon honey or agave syrup (optional)

Instructions:

- Spoon cottage cheese into a bowl.
- Arrange sliced fresh fruit on top of the cottage cheese.
- Sprinkle chopped nuts over the fruit, if using.
- Drizzle with honey or agave syrup for added sweetness, if desired.

- Enjoy this protein-packed snack that's both satisfying and nutritious.

13.   Shrimp Stir-Fry with Vegetables

Ingredients:

- 8 oz raw shrimp, peeled and deveined
- 2 cups mixed vegetables (such as bell peppers, snap peas, carrots, and broccoli)
- 2 cloves garlic, minced
- 1 tablespoon low-sodium soy sauce
- 1 tablespoon hoisin sauce
- 1 teaspoon sesame oil
- Cooked brown rice or quinoa, for serving

Instructions:

- Heat sesame oil in a large skillet or wok over medium-high heat.
- Add minced garlic to the skillet and cook until fragrant, about 30 seconds.
- Add raw shrimp to the skillet and stir-fry until pink and opaque, about 2-3 minutes.
- Add mixed vegetables to the skillet and stir-fry until crisp-tender, about 3-4 minutes.
- In a small bowl, whisk together soy sauce and hoisin sauce. Pour the sauce over the shrimp and vegetables in the skillet.
- Cook for an additional 1-2 minutes, stirring constantly, until the sauce thickens and coats the shrimp and vegetables.

- Serve the shrimp stir-fry over cooked brown rice or quinoa for a flavorful and satisfying dinner.

14. Chocolate Banana Smoothie

Ingredients:

- 1 ripe banana, peeled and sliced
- 1 tablespoon unsweetened cocoa powder
- 1/2 cup low-tyramine milk alternative (such as almond milk or coconut milk)
- 1/2 cup plain Greek yogurt (low-tyramine)
- 1 tablespoon honey or maple syrup (optional)
- Ice cubes

Instructions:

- Place sliced banana, cocoa powder, low-tyramine milk alternative, plain Greek yogurt, and honey or maple syrup (if using) in a blender.
- Add a handful of ice cubes to the blender.
- Blend on high speed until smooth and creamy.
- Pour the smoothie into glasses and serve immediately

15. Greek Yogurt Parfait with Nutty Granola

Ingredients:

- 1/2 cup plain Greek yogurt (low-tyramine)
- 1/4 cup homemade or store-bought low-tyramine granola
- 1/4 cup mixed fresh berries (such as raspberries, blueberries, or strawberries)
- 1 tablespoon honey or agave syrup (optional)
- 1 tablespoon chopped nuts (such as almonds or walnuts)

Instructions:

- In a glass or bowl, layer plain Greek yogurt, low-tyramine granola, and mixed fresh berries.
- Drizzle honey or agave syrup over the layers for added sweetness, if desired.
- Sprinkle chopped nuts on top for extra crunch and flavor.
- Repeat the layers if desired, ending with a layer of granola and berries on top.
- Serve immediately as a nutritious and satisfying breakfast option.

16.   Caprese Salad with Balsamic Glaze

Ingredients:

- 1 large ripe tomato, sliced
- 4 oz fresh mozzarella cheese, sliced
- Fresh basil leaves
- 1 tablespoon balsamic glaze
- Salt and pepper to taste

Instructions:

- Arrange alternating slices of tomato and mozzarella cheese on a plate or platter.
- Tuck fresh basil leaves between the slices of tomato and cheese.
- Drizzle balsamic glaze over the salad.
- Season with salt and pepper to taste.
- Serve immediately as a refreshing and light lunch option.

17. Turkey Meatballs with Zucchini Noodles

Ingredients:

- 1 lb lean ground turkey
- 1/4 cup breadcrumbs (made from low-tyramine bread)
- 1 egg
- 2 cloves garlic, minced
- 2 tablespoons chopped fresh parsley
- Salt and pepper to taste
- 2 medium zucchini, spiralized into noodles
- 1 cup marinara sauce (low-tyramine)
- Grated Parmesan cheese (optional)

Instructions:

- Preheat oven to 375°F (190°C). Line a baking sheet with parchment paper.
- In a large bowl, combine ground turkey, breadcrumbs, egg, minced garlic, chopped fresh parsley, salt, and pepper. Mix until well combined.

- Shape the turkey mixture into meatballs and place them on the prepared baking sheet.
- Bake meatballs in the preheated oven for 20-25 minutes, or until cooked through and browned.
- While the meatballs are baking, heat marinara sauce in a large skillet over medium heat. Add zucchini noodles and cook until tender, about 3-5 minutes.
- Serve turkey meatballs over zucchini noodles with marinara sauce. Sprinkle with grated Parmesan cheese, if desired, before serving.

18. Mango Coconut Chia Pudding

Ingredients:

- 1 ripe mango, peeled and diced
- 1 cup low-tyramine milk alternative (such as coconut milk or almond milk)
- 1/4 cup chia seeds
- 1 tablespoon honey or maple syrup (optional)
- Shredded coconut for garnish (optional)

Instructions:

- In a blender, combine diced mango and low-tyramine milk alternative. Blend until smooth.
- Transfer the mango mixture to a bowl or jar. Stir in chia seeds and honey or maple syrup (if using).
- Cover and refrigerate for at least 4 hours or overnight, until the chia pudding thickens.

- Serve chilled, topped with shredded coconut for garnish if desired.

19.   Stuffed Bell Peppers

Ingredients:

- 2 bell peppers (any color), halved and seeds removed
- 1/2 cup cooked quinoa
- 1/2 cup black beans, drained and rinsed
- 1/4 cup diced tomatoes
- 1/4 cup diced avocado
- 1/4 cup shredded cheddar cheese (optional)
- 1 tablespoon chopped fresh cilantro
- Salt and pepper to taste

Instructions:

- Preheat the oven to 375°F (190°C). Place the bell pepper halves on a baking sheet.
- In a bowl, mix together cooked quinoa, black beans, diced tomatoes, diced avocado, shredded cheddar cheese (if using), chopped cilantro, salt, and pepper.
- Spoon the quinoa mixture into each bell pepper half until filled.
- Bake in the preheated oven for 20-25 minutes, or until the peppers are tender and the filling is heated through.
- Serve as a nutritious and satisfying snack or light meal.

20.   Baked Cod with Lemon and Herbs

Ingredients:

- 2 cod fillets
- 2 tablespoons olive oil
- 1 tablespoon lemon juice
- 2 cloves garlic, minced
- 1 teaspoon dried thyme
- 1 teaspoon dried parsley
- Salt and pepper to taste
- Lemon slices for garnish

Instructions:

- Preheat the oven to 375°F (190°C). Place the cod fillets on a baking sheet lined with parchment paper.
- In a small bowl, whisk together olive oil, lemon juice, minced garlic, dried thyme, dried parsley, salt, and pepper.
- Brush the olive oil mixture over the cod fillets, coating them evenly.
- Place a lemon slice on top of each fillet for garnish.
- Bake in the preheated oven for 15-20 minutes, or until the cod is opaque and flakes easily with a fork.
- Serve hot with your choice of side dishes, such as steamed vegetables or a mixed green salad.

21.   Apple Cinnamon Baked Oatmeal

Ingredients:

- 2 cups rolled oats
- 1 1/2 cups low-tyramine milk alternative (such as almond milk or oat milk)
- 1/4 cup maple syrup
- 1 teaspoon vanilla extract
- 1 teaspoon ground cinnamon
- 1/4 teaspoon ground nutmeg
- 1 apple, peeled and diced
- 1/4 cup chopped nuts (such as walnuts or pecans)
- 1 tablespoon melted coconut oil
- Pinch of salt

Instructions:

- Preheat the oven to 375°F (190°C). Grease a baking dish with coconut oil.
- In a large bowl, combine rolled oats, low-tyramine milk alternative, maple syrup, vanilla extract, ground cinnamon, ground nutmeg, diced apple, chopped nuts, melted coconut oil, and a pinch of salt.
- Pour the oatmeal mixture into the prepared baking dish, spreading it out evenly.
- Bake in the preheated oven for 35-40 minutes, or until the top is golden brown and the oats are cooked through.
- Serve warm, optionally topped with a drizzle of maple syrup or a dollop of yogurt.

22.   Banana Oatmeal

Ingredients:

- 1/2 cup rolled oats
- 1 cup water or low-tyramine milk alternative
- 1 ripe banana, mashed
- 1 tablespoon honey or maple syrup (optional)
- Pinch of cinnamon (optional)

Instructions:

- In a small saucepan, bring water or milk to a boil.
- Stir in rolled oats and reduce heat to low. Cook for 5-7 minutes, stirring occasionally, until oats are tender and creamy.
- Remove from heat and stir in mashed banana, honey or maple syrup, and cinnamon, if using.
- Serve hot, garnished with additional banana slices or nuts if desired.

23.   Lemon Herb Roasted Chicken

Ingredients:

- 4 bone-in, skin-on chicken thighs
- 2 tablespoons olive oil
- 2 cloves garlic, minced
- 1 tablespoon chopped fresh parsley
- 1 tablespoon chopped fresh thyme
- 1 tablespoon chopped fresh rosemary
- Zest and juice of 1 lemon

- Salt and pepper to taste

Instructions:

- Preheat the oven to 400°F (200°C).
- In a small bowl, whisk together olive oil, minced garlic, chopped fresh parsley, chopped fresh thyme, chopped fresh rosemary, lemon zest, lemon juice, salt, and pepper to make the marinade.
- Place the chicken thighs in a baking dish and pour the marinade over them, turning to coat evenly.
- Arrange the chicken thighs skin-side up in the baking dish.
- Roast in the preheated oven for 30-35 minutes, or until the chicken is cooked through and the skin is crispy and golden brown.
- Remove from the oven and let rest for a few minutes before serving.

24.   Chocolate Avocado Mousse

Ingredients:

- 2 ripe avocados, peeled and pitted
- 1/4 cup unsweetened cocoa powder
- 1/4 cup honey or maple syrup
- 1 teaspoon vanilla extract
- Pinch of salt
- Fresh berries for serving (optional)

Instructions:

- In a food processor or blender, combine ripe avocados, unsweetened cocoa powder, honey or maple syrup, vanilla extract, and a pinch of salt.
- Blend until smooth and creamy, scraping down the sides of the bowl as needed.
- Transfer the chocolate avocado mousse to serving bowls or glasses.
- Refrigerate for at least 30 minutes to chill before serving.
- Serve chilled, garnished with fresh berries if desired.

25.   Banana Nut Overnight Oats

Ingredients:

- 1/2 cup rolled oats
- 1/2 cup low-tyramine milk alternative (such as almond milk or soy milk)
- 1/2 ripe banana, mashed
- 1 tablespoon chopped nuts (such as almonds, walnuts, or pecans)
- 1 tablespoon maple syrup or honey
- 1/2 teaspoon ground cinnamon

Instructions:

- In a mason jar or container, combine rolled oats, low-tyramine milk alternative, mashed banana, chopped nuts, maple syrup or honey, and ground cinnamon.
- Stir well to combine all ingredients.

- Cover the jar with a lid and refrigerate overnight, or for at least 4 hours.

26.   Quinoa and Black Bean Salad

Ingredients:

- 1 cup cooked quinoa, cooled
- 1 can (15 oz) black beans, drained and rinsed
- 1/2 cup diced bell pepper (any color)
- 1/4 cup diced red onion
- 1/4 cup chopped fresh cilantro
- Juice of 1 lime
- 2 tablespoons extra virgin olive oil
- Salt and pepper to taste

Instructions:

- In a large mixing bowl, combine cooked quinoa, black beans, diced bell pepper, diced red onion, and chopped fresh cilantro.
- In a small bowl, whisk together lime juice, extra virgin olive oil, salt, and pepper to make the dressing.
- Pour the dressing over the quinoa and black bean salad and toss until well coated.
- Refrigerate the salad for at least 30 minutes to allow the flavors to meld before serving.
- Serve chilled as a nutritious and satisfying lunch option.

Grilled Salmon with Asparagus

Ingredients:

- 2 salmon fillets
- 1 tablespoon olive oil
- 1 teaspoon lemon zest
- 1 tablespoon lemon juice
- 2 cloves garlic, minced
- 1 teaspoon dried dill
- Salt and pepper to taste
- 1 bunch asparagus, trimmed

Instructions:

- Preheat the grill to medium-high heat.
- In a small bowl, whisk together olive oil, lemon zest, lemon juice, minced garlic, dried dill, salt, and pepper to make the marinade.
- Place the salmon fillets in a shallow dish and pour the marinade over them, turning to coat evenly. Let marinate for 15-30 minutes.
- Meanwhile, toss the trimmed asparagus with a drizzle of olive oil, salt, and pepper.
- Grill the salmon fillets for 4-5 minutes per side, or until cooked through and flaky.
- During the last few minutes of grilling the salmon, add the asparagus to the grill and cook until tender-crisp, about 3-4 minutes per side.
- Serve the grilled salmon and asparagus hot with a squeeze of lemon juice.

28.   **Raspberry Chia Seed Pudding**

Ingredients:

- 1 cup low-tyramine milk alternative (such as coconut milk or almond milk)
- 1/4 cup chia seeds
- 1 tablespoon honey or maple syrup
- 1/2 teaspoon vanilla extract
- 1/2 cup fresh raspberries

Instructions:

- In a mixing bowl, whisk together low-tyramine milk alternative, chia seeds, honey or maple syrup, and vanilla extract until well combined.
- Gently fold in fresh raspberries.
- Transfer the mixture to serving bowls or glasses.
- Cover and refrigerate for at least 2 hours, or until the chia seed pudding thickens.
- Serve chilled, optionally topped with additional fresh raspberries.

29.   **Veggie Egg Muffins**

Ingredients:

- 6 eggs

- 1/4 cup diced bell peppers
- 1/4 cup diced tomatoes
- 1/4 cup diced onions
- 1/4 cup chopped spinach
- 1/4 cup shredded cheese (optional)
- Salt and pepper to taste

Instructions:

- Preheat the oven to 350°F (175°C) and grease a muffin tin with cooking spray.
- In a mixing bowl, whisk together eggs, diced bell peppers, diced tomatoes, diced onions, chopped spinach, shredded cheese (if using), salt, and pepper.
- Pour the egg mixture evenly into the prepared muffin tin, filling each cup about 3/4 full.
- Bake in the preheated oven for 20-25 minutes, or until the egg muffins are set and lightly golden on top.
- Allow the egg muffins to cool slightly before removing them from the muffin tin. Serve warm or store in the refrigerator for later use.

30.   Turkey Avocado Wrap

Ingredients:

- 2 large whole wheat or low-tyramine wraps
- 4 slices deli turkey
- 1/2 avocado, sliced
- 1/4 cup shredded lettuce

- 1/4 cup diced tomatoes
- 2 tablespoons hummus
- Salt and pepper to taste

Instructions:

- Lay the wraps flat on a clean surface.
- Spread 1 tablespoon of hummus onto each wrap.
- Divide the sliced turkey, avocado slices, shredded lettuce, and diced tomatoes between the two wraps.
- Season with salt and pepper to taste.
- Roll up the wraps tightly, tucking in the sides as you go.
- Cut each wrap in half diagonally and serve immediately, or wrap them tightly in foil or parchment paper for later.

31. Veggie Stir-Fry with Tofu

Ingredients:

- 1 block extra firm tofu, drained and cubed
- 2 tablespoons soy sauce
- 1 tablespoon sesame oil
- 1 tablespoon olive oil
- 2 cloves garlic, minced
- 1 tablespoon grated ginger
- 2 cups mixed vegetables (such as broccoli, bell peppers, snap peas, carrots)
- Cooked rice or noodles, for serving

Instructions:

- In a bowl, toss the cubed tofu with soy sauce and sesame oil until well coated. Let marinate for 10-15 minutes.
- Heat olive oil in a large skillet or wok over medium-high heat.
- Add minced garlic and grated ginger to the skillet and cook until fragrant, about 30 seconds.
- Add the marinated tofu to the skillet and cook until golden brown on all sides, about 5-7 minutes.
- Add mixed vegetables to the skillet and stir-fry until crisp-tender, about 3-5 minutes.
- Serve the tofu and vegetable stir-fry hot over cooked rice or noodles.

32. Mixed Berry Smoothie Bowl

Ingredients:

- 1 cup mixed berries (such as strawberries, blueberries, raspberries)
- 1/2 banana, sliced
- 1/2 cup low-tyramine milk alternative (such as almond milk or coconut milk)
- 1 tablespoon honey or maple syrup
- Toppings: sliced banana, fresh berries, granola, shredded coconut, chia seeds

Instructions:

- In a blender, combine mixed berries, sliced banana, low-tyramine milk alternative, and honey or maple syrup. Blend until smooth.

- Pour the smoothie into a bowl.
- Top with sliced banana, fresh berries, granola, shredded coconut, and chia seeds.
- Serve immediately and enjoy with a spoon.

33.   Peanut Butter Banana Smoothie

Ingredients:

- 1 ripe banana
- 2 tablespoons peanut butter (check for low-tyramine options)
- 1 cup low-tyramine milk alternative (such as almond milk or soy milk)
- 1 tablespoon honey or maple syrup
- 1/2 teaspoon vanilla extract
- Handful of ice cubes

Instructions:

- In a blender, combine the ripe banana, peanut butter, low-tyramine milk alternative, honey or maple syrup, vanilla extract, and ice cubes.
- Blend until smooth and creamy.
- Pour into glasses and serve immediately as a delicious and nutritious breakfast smoothie.

34.   Greek Chickpea Salad

Ingredients:

- 1 can (15 oz) chickpeas, drained and rinsed
- 1 cucumber, diced
- 1 bell pepper, diced
- 1/4 cup red onion, thinly sliced
- 1/4 cup Kalamata olives, pitted and halved
- 1/4 cup crumbled feta cheese (optional)
- 2 tablespoons chopped fresh parsley
- 2 tablespoons extra virgin olive oil
- 1 tablespoon red wine vinegar
- 1 teaspoon dried oregano
- Salt and pepper to taste

Instructions:

- In a large mixing bowl, combine the chickpeas, diced cucumber, diced bell pepper, thinly sliced red onion, halved Kalamata olives, crumbled feta cheese (if using), and chopped fresh parsley.
- In a small bowl, whisk together the extra virgin olive oil, red wine vinegar, dried oregano, salt, and pepper to make the dressing.
- Pour the dressing over the chickpea salad and toss until well coated.
- Refrigerate the salad for at least 30 minutes to allow the flavors to meld before serving.
- Serve chilled as a refreshing and satisfying lunch option.

35.   Vanilla cupcakes with fudgy frosting

INGREDIENTS

Vanilla cupcakes

- 2 eggs
- 2 cups all-purpose flour (gluten-free) Bob's Red Mill 1-to-1 is best (includes xanthan gum)
- 1-1/2 teaspoons psyllium husk powder (only if using a flour blend that doesn't include xanthan gum)
- 2-1/2 teaspoons baking powder
- 1/2 teaspoon baking soda
- 3/4 cup agave syrup honey, or maple syrup
- 3/4 cup coconut milk whole milk, hemp milk, rice milk
- 1/3 cup grapeseed oil sunflower seed oil, light olive oil
- 2 tablespoons vanilla extract alcohol-free for migraine diet

Fudgy frosting

- 1 cup coconut sugar (organic)
- 1 cup sweet potato puree (canned or use a baked sweet potato)
- 40 drops stevia (organic) drops, vanilla flavor preferred
- 4 teaspoons vanilla extract alcohol-free for migraine diet
- 1/2 cup carob powder
- 1/2 cup carob chips Sunspire brand unsweeted carob chips
- 1/2 cup tahini or unsalted sunflower seed butter
- 1/4 cup coconut oil

INSTRUCTIONS

Vanilla cupcakes

- Preheat oven to 350F/180C/gas mark 4. Line 18 cupcake tins with liners.
- Separate the eggs.
- Beat egg whites until stiff peaks form. Set aside.
- In a medium bowl, whisk flour with baking powder, baking soda, and psyllium husk powder (if using).
- In a mixing bowl (or the bowl of a stand mixer), beat egg yolks, agave syrup, coconut milk, oil, and vanilla until smooth.
- Add flour mixture and beat just until no lumps remain. Fold in egg whites using a spatula until mixed in completely.
- Scoop batter into prepared pans, about 2/3 full. Place on center rack. Bake 10 minutes, then rotate pans. Bake another 10 minutes, or until tops spring back and a toothpick comes out clean.
- Cool completely on wire racks before frosting.

Fudgy frosting

- Place coconut sugar in blender and blend on high for one minute or until a fine powder.
- Place sweet potato and stevia in food processor fitted with S-blade. Process until smooth.
- In a heavy-bottomed saucepan, place remaining ingredients and stir over low-medium heat until melted and smooth. Scrape into food processor. Blend until very smooth.
- For thick fudgy frosting, immediately spread on cupcakes. For pipe-able buttercream style frosting, refrigerate until cold. Then beat until fluffy. Use a large piping tip to create frosting swirls as shown.

INGREDIENTS

- 8 cups chicken stock (low-sodium) homemade or store-bought
- 3 bay leaves
- 5 sprigs thyme (fresh)
- 3 sprigs fennel optional (it grows in my garden)
- 1 chicken breast skin-on, bone-in preferred
- 1 chicken back optional, for flavor
- 3 carrots thickly sliced
- 3 potatoes organic gold, medium-sized, large dice
- 5 stalks celery thickly sliced
- 1 bundle Italian flat-leaf parsley (fresh) finely chopped

INSTRUCTIONS

- Bring the chicken stock just to barely a boil in a large heavy soup pot.
- Tie the herbs together with kitchen string and add to the pot with the chicken breast and chicken back if using.
- Make sure the stock doesn't boil, if you have an instant-read thermometer you are looking for the temperature of the liquid to be 180F/82C.
- Prep the vegetables while the chicken is cooking.
- Poach the chicken for up to 30 minutes, or until chicken is cooked. It should be 165F/75C inside. Use tongs to remove

chicken and herb bundle, setting chicken to cool on a cutting board and composting the herb bundle.

- Turn up the heat to just barely boiling, add the vegetables and cook until fork tender, about 10 minutes. Turn off the heat.
- Once chicken is cool enough to handle, remove skin, bones, and cartilage (saving in the freezer for a future pot of stock), and dice.
- Add chicken to soup. Ladle soup into bowls and stir about 2 tbsp chopped parsley into each serving.
- You can add the remaining parsley to the soup and store in the fridge, or leave it separate and add just before serving hot soup.

37.   Granola

INGREDIENTS

- 2 cups rolled oats (gluten-free) gluten-free (200 g)
- 1 cup coconut (flakes, unsweetened) (50 g)
- 1 cup pumpkin seeds raw, pepitas (120 g)
- 1 cup sunflower seeds raw (130 g)
- 1 cup walnuts hazelnuts, pecans, raw (115 g) (omit for migraine diet)
- 1 tbsp olive oil (extra virgin)
- 1/2 tsp cinnamon
- 1/4 cup maple syrup (omit for migraine diet)
- 1/4 tsp sea salt (omit for very low sodium diets)
- 1 cup raisins (160 g) (omit for migraine diet)

INSTRUCTIONS

- Preheat oven to 300F/150C/gas mark 2. Spray a rimmed baking sheet that's lined with parchment paper with cooking spray.
- In a large bowl, whisk the olive oil, cinnamon, maple syrup, and salt.
- Add all the other ingredients except the raisins or dried fruit and toss well to coat.
- Pour out onto the baking sheet and put in the oven for 15 minutes.
- Stir, then set the time for another 10 minutes and check it.
- Bake for up to 30 minutes total. You want it to be golden brown but not too crispy.
- Once cool, add the raisins or dried fruit and mix well.
- Once completely cool, store in an airtight container for up to 3 week

38.   Wild rice and carrots

INGREDIENTS

- 1 handful Italian flat-leaf parsley (fresh)
- 1 cup wild rice (150 g)
- 1 tablespoon olive oil (extra virgin) unsalted butter
- 2 carrots large
- 2 ribs celery
- 1/2 teaspoon black pepper

- Wash the parsley and roll up in a towel.
- Rinse and drain the rice, then add 2 C. (500 ml) filtered water or unsalted chicken or vegetable stock. Cover and bring to a boil in a medium saucepan, then turn down the heat to low and cook for 45 minutes. Turn off the heat and leave the cover on for at least 10 minutes.
- When the rice is done, scrub the carrots and slice very thinly on the diagonal.
- Wash the celery and finely mince.
- Finely chop the parsley.
- Heat olive oil or butter in a large skillet over medium heat. Add carrot and celery; cook 6-8 minutes or until tender, stirring frequently. Stir in rice, parsley, and pepper.
- Cook one minute until everything is warmed through.

39.   Vegetarian Fried Quinoa

Ingredients

- Stir Fry
- 1 cup dry quinoa
- 2 cups vegetable broth
- 1 teaspoon sesame oil
- 2 Japanese eggplants, chopped
- 2 zucchini, wash and chopped into ½" pieces
- 5 carrots, chopped
- 1 red pepper, chopped

- 6 oz mushrooms
- 1 bunch of green onions, trimmed at the ends and chopped
- Sesame Sauce
- 1 cup coconut aminos
- 6 tablespoon tahini
- 2 teaspoon distilled white vinegar
- 2 teaspoon toasted sesame oil
- 4 cloves garlic, peeled and minced
- 4 teaspoon ground mustard
- 2 teaspoon fresh ginger, peeled and grated
- kosher salt and pepper to taste

Instructions

- For the sauce - Add all the ingredients to a food processor and blend till combined. Set aside.
- Cook quinoa according to package with vegetable broth. I use Bob's Red Mill because it is already rinsed. Most others need to be rinsed first.
- Add sesame oil to a skillet or wok on high heat. Add all the veggies except for 2 green onion and toss. The veggies should take about 3-4 minutes to cook. You still want them a little crisp. (I use Japanese eggplant because it doesn't need to be peeled, has less seeds, is less bitter and a little creamier, but any eggplant will work)
- Add the cooked quinoa to the skillet and toss everything together with the sauce. Serve and top with the 2 chopped green onions.

 Spicy Kale & Swiss Chard Saute

INGREDIENTS

- 1 tablespoon extra virgin coconut oil, or ghee
- 1 bunch green onions, thinly sliced
- 3 cloves garlic, minced
- 1 jalapeño, thinly sliced (optional)
- 1 bunch Swiss Chard, 500g, stems & leaves removed, thinly sliced
- 1 bunch Kale, 500g, stems and leaves thinly sliced
- 1 tablespoon hot sesame oil
- 1 tablespoon dark toasted sesame oil
- 1 tablespoon raw sunflower seeds
- 1 tablespoon raw pumpkin seeds
- 1 tablespoon raw sesame seeds

INSTRUCTIONS

- In a large frying pan or sauté pan set over medium–high heat, melt the coconut oil. Add the onions, garlic, and jalapeño, if using, and sauté for 5 minutes, or until golden.
- Add the chard stems and cook for another 3 to 4 minutes. Add the rest of the chard and the kale. Cover the pan with a lid to help the greens wilt, about 5 minutes. Once they have wilted a bit, add the hot and dark toasted sesame oils, stirring to coat.
- Add the sunflower, pumpkin, and sesame seeds and continue to sauté, uncovered, for 10 minutes, or until cooked through.

41.   Sauer kraut

INGREDIENTS

- 1 head cabbage green or red
- 3-4 carrots large
- 1 bulb fennel
- 1-2 tbsp sea salt kosher salt

INSTRUCTIONS

- Wash the vegetables.
- Set a large bowl on the counter, with the salt next to it. As you shred the veggies, add them to the bowl. Sprinkle each layer lightly with salt. (You can make this without salt, although it will not be as crispy.)
- Remove any wilted outer leaves, then cut the cabbage in quarters and remove the hard core. Using a sharp knife or a food processor fitted with a shredder disk, shred or finely slice the cabbage.
- Shred or grate the carrots.
- Remove any hard stems from the fennel, then finely chop.
- Mix everything together thoroughly. The salt draws the water out of the vegetables and creates a natural brine.
- Pack the crock, using the flat-bottomed cup to mash each layer flat, removing any air. Once you have all the vegetables in there, put the plate on top and press down. You should already have a fair bit of brine (salty liquid). Add the weight. Press again.
- You need to have the liquid rise above the level of the plate, so that the vegetables are not in contact with air (otherwise

you will get mold, not fermentation). This usually happens within a few hours. If it hasn't happened overnight, then make 1 cup of salt water by mixing 1 T. (5 g) of salt with 1 C. (250 ml) of filtered water and pour it in.

- Put a clean kitchen towel over the crock. This allows air to do its magic while keeping insects and dust out. Place the crock in a cool dark place. I check it after 3 or 4 days, and skim off any foam that has formed, washing the rock, then replacing it.
- I taste it after 5 days, sometimes 7 if I forget. Putting a sticky-note on my kitchen calendar helps me remember when I started it.
- That's it! Once the kraut is ready, remove it to a container and store it in the refrigerator.

42.　　Golden bell pepper soup

INGREDIENTS

- 1/4 cup olive oil (extra virgin)
- 1/2 onions small, diced
- 2 carrots medium, peeled and diced
- 1 stalk celery diced
- 8 bell peppers (capsicum) red, yellow, or orange
- 1 sweet potatoes large, peeled and chopped
- 4 cups vegetable stock (low-sodium)
- 3 tsp marjoram (fresh) finely chopped

INSTRUCTIONS

- In a large pot, heat the oil over medium heat.
- Add the onion, carrot, celery, and a pinch of sea salt and black pepper.
- Cook until the vegetables are tender, about 4 minutes.
- Add the bell peppers and cook until soft, about 6 minutes.
- Add the sweet potatoes and broth. Season with sea salt and black pepper, cover the pot, and bring to a boil.
- Lower the heat and add the marjoram. Simmer until the vegetables are tender, about 20 minutes.
- Let the soup cool slightly, and then, in batches, transfer to a blender and puree until smooth. If needed, thin the soup with water.
- Adjust the seasoning with sea salt and black pepper if necessary.
- Return the soup to the pot to keep warm until serving.
- Serve garnished with the Herbed Croutons and, if desired, the avocado and cilantro on top and Seriously Sensational Sriracha Sauce on the side.

43.   taco salad

INGREDIENTS

Creamy spicy dressing

- 2 ounces hemp seeds (1/2 cup) raw, soaked for at least 4 hours
- 2 tbsp olive oil (extra virgin)
- 2 tbsp water (filtered or spring)

- 1 tbsp white vinegar use lemon juice if not on the migraine diet
- 1 clove garlic
- 1/2 tsp white pepper
- 1/2 tsp smoked paprika (pimenton)
- 1/2 tsp cumin (dried)
- 1 sprig Italian flat-leaf parsley (fresh) or cilantro
- 4 small cherry tomatoes
- Taco seasoning
- 2 tbsp chili powder preferably California chili powder
- 2 tbsp smoked paprika (pimenton)
- 1 tbsp cumin (dried)
- 1 tbsp garlic powder
- 1 tbsp onion powder (omit for migraine diet)
- 1/2 tsp oregano (dried)
- 1/4 tsp chipotle powder or cayenne

Salad

- 16 ounces beef (grass-fed) ground (see above for vegan substitutes)
- 2 bell peppers (capsicum), red and yellow, thinly sliced
- 2 onions (green) scallions, spring onions, sliced on the diagonal
- 4 cups romaine lettuce salad greens, spring mix
- 1 pint cherry tomatoes
- 1 avocado
- 3 radishes thinly sliced, or jicama cut into sticks

INSTRUCTIONS

Creamy spicy dressing

- Soak the hemp seeds in filtered water for at least four hours. Drain and rinse thoroughly.
- Place all dressing ingredients in the blender and blend until smooth and creamy. Set aside.
- Taco seasoning
- Mix all ingredients together until one color. This makes enough for two recipes.

Salad

- Heat a cast-iron skillet over medium-high heat. Add the beef, breaking up with a spoon and cooking until no longer pink.
- Sprinkle 3 tbsp taco seasoning evenly over the beef and add one cup (200 ml) of filtered water. Stir to mix thoroughly. Continue to cook over medium heat until the moisture is gone and beef is cooked. Remove beef to a warm plate. Do not wipe out the pan.

- Add 1 tbsp (15 ml) coconut oil, extra-virgin olive oil, or rendered bacon fat to the pan, tilting to coat evenly.
- Sauté the peppers and the green onion for 10 minutes until golden and fairly limp.
- To serve as shown, lay out ingredients on a large platter with the dressing on the side.

44.   Berry crepes with ricotta cheese

INGREDIENTS

- Crepes
- 1/3 cup sweet sorghum flour (45 g)
- 1/4 cup tapioca flour (40 g)
- 1/4 cup brown rice flour (40 g)
- 1/4 cup teff flour or seeds (49 g)
- 1 cup milk organic, or half and half
- 1/4 cup water (filtered or spring)
- 3 eggs
- 3 tbsp butter (unsalted) organic or Kerrygold
- Vanilla ricotta cream
- 15 ounces ricotta (whole-milk) organic
- 1 tbsp vanilla extract
- 1/2 tsp cinnamon Vietnamese if possible
- 1/8-1/4 tsp nutmeg (dried) freshly ground
- 2-3 packets stevia (organic) Pyure brand

INSTRUCTIONS

- Crepes
- Put the first four ingredients in the blender and blend until a fine powder.
- Add milk, water, and eggs and blend for one minute. Let stand at least 20 minutes, 30 is better.
- Melt the butter and blend in just before cooking the crepes.
- Heat a non-stick large skillet or frying pan over medium heat. No oil is needed; there is enough in the batter.
- Pulse once or twice to remix, each time, before pouring 1/4 cup of batter into the center of the pan, tilting it in a circle to spread the batter into a thin circle.

- Cook two minutes until just set, then flip with a spatula or tongs, and cook another 30 seconds.
- Remove to a plate, then pour the next crepe. I fill the ones we are going to eat while each is cooking, putting them on another plate.
- Stuff with ricotta cream and berries.
- Cool extra crepes on separate plates (they stick together), then stack, separated by waxed paper, and wrap with plastic wrap, in a heavy freezer-safe bag to freeze. They are also great for dinner.
- Vanilla ricotta cream
- Mix together in a bowl, then replace back in the tub for storage. Eat within four days.
- To fill crepes, put into a zip-top bag, close, then snip off a corner and use it to pipe the cream into each crepe.

45.   Waakye

INGREDIENTS

- 1 cup black-eyed peas dried
- 3 cups vegetable stock (low-sodium) see my Notes below
- 2 tbsp coconut oil
- 1/2 cup onions yellow, chopped
- 2 cloves garlic minced
- 1 cup white rice long-grain, such as Carolina Gold, rinsed and drained 6 times
- 2 bay leaves
- 1/2 tsp baking soda
- 1/2 tsp kosher salt

- Pick through the dried peas, removing any stones, twigs, or unhappy-looking beans. Soak in filtered water overnight, adding more to the bowl if the beans absorb it all. Rinse and drain well.
- Put the beans in a large pot with a tight-fitting lid, add the vegetable stock, and place over high heat. Bring to a boil, then turn the heat down to low and simmer, uncovered, for 30-40 minutes.
- After the black-eyed peas are tender, heat the coconut oil in a skillet over medium-high heat. Add the onion and garlic and sauté until the onion is translucent, about 5 minutes, stirring as needed.
- Add the onion mixture to the large pot with the remaining ingredients, stirring well.
- Return the pot to a boil, then turn down to a low simmer and cook, covered, until the rice and beans are tender, about 30 minutes.

46.   Veggie quiche cups

INGREDIENTS

- 10 ounces broccoli chopped, or other vegetable finely chopped
- 4 eggs pastured, free range
- 3/4 cup ricotta (whole-milk) whole-milk (180 g)
- 1/2 cup bell peppers red, orange, yellow, finely diced (60 g)

- 1 onions (green) scallions, spring onions (20 g)
- 3 drops hot sauce
- 1/2 tsp black pepper

- INSTRUCTIONS
- If using frozen vegetables, microwave for 2-3 minutes on high until thawed. Squeeze dry with your hands or a food press (or else the quiches won't set).
- Line a 12-cup muffin pan with 8 foil baking cups or place 8 silicone cups on a baking sheet. Spray with cooking spray if using foil cups.
- Preheat oven to 350F/180C/gas mark 4.
- Blend all ingredients together in a bowl, mixing well. Divide evenly among the cups.
- Bake for 30 minutes until they feel firm to the touch in the center (you may still see some bubbling, but they will set as they cool).
- Let cool on wire rack. Wrap extras in plastic wrap once cool and store in a freezer-safe bag.

47.　　Lemon Herb Baked Cod

Ingredients:

- 4 cod fillets
- 2 tablespoons olive oil
- 2 cloves garlic, minced
- Zest and juice of 1 lemon

- 1 tablespoon chopped fresh parsley
- 1 tablespoon chopped fresh dill
- Salt and pepper to taste

Instructions:

- Preheat the oven to 400°F (200°C). Line a baking dish with parchment paper.
- Place the cod fillets in the prepared baking dish.
- In a small bowl, whisk together the olive oil, minced garlic, lemon zest, lemon juice, chopped fresh parsley, chopped fresh dill, salt, and pepper.
- Pour the lemon herb mixture over the cod fillets, coating them evenly.
- Bake in the preheated oven for 12-15 minutes, or until the cod is opaque and flakes easily with a fork.
- Serve the lemon herb baked cod hot with your choice of side dishes.

48.   Comforting roasted tomato soup

Ingredients

- 2 pounds tomatoes seeded and cored, preferably farmer's market tomatoes
- 1 tablespoon olive oil (extra virgin)

- 6 sprigs thyme (fresh) washed and lightly dried in a towel
- 1 tablespoons butter (unsalted) or buttery spread for plant-based version
- 1/4 cup heavy cream (organic) or coconut cream for dairy-free/vegan/paleo version
- 1/4 cup chicken stock (low-sodium) or vegetable stock for plant-based version
- 1/4 teaspoon black pepper freshly cracked
- 1/4 teaspoon sea salt omit for lower-sodium version

Instructions

- Preheat oven to 425ºF /220C/gas mark 6.5.
- Place tomatoes in a baking dish and drizzle with olive oil, a little sea salt and pepper, and the thyme sprigs. Roast for 45 minutes. Remove thyme sprigs.
- Spoon tomatoes into the blender and add remaining ingredients. Blend until smooth. Serve immediately.

49.   Curried pumpkin and red lentil soup with vegan sour cream

Ingredients

- Curried pumpkin and red lentil soup
- 1-1/2 cups lentils red (270 g)
- 3 cups vegetable stock (low-sodium)
- 15 ounces pumpkin purée
- 1-1/2 tsp curry powder mild or medium
- 1 tsp smoked salt
- Vegan sour cream
- 1/2 cup cashews raw (60 g)
- 1/2 lemons
- 1/2 tsp sea salt

Instructions

- Soak the cashews in enough filtered water to completely cover them while you are making the soup.
- Rinse the lentils after checking them to remove any debris (like small pebbles or bits of dried plants). Drain the lentils, then put them in a soup pot with the vegetable stock, pumpkin, curry powder, and smoked salt. Bring to a boil and cook for 30 minutes, or until the lentils are tender. Turn off the heat.
- Drain the soaked cashews and put them into your blender with the juice from the lemon half and the salt. Blend, stopping to scrape down the sides as needed. (Use the tamper if you have a Vitamix.) The mixture should end up a very smooth sour cream consistency. If you need to, add a little bit of filtered water to get it to blend.
- Scrape out the cashew mixture into a storage bowl. DO NOT WASH THE BLENDER.

- Add the soup mixture to the blender and hold down the lid with a kitchen towel. Gradually bring up the speed on the blender so you don't create too much hot steam. Blend until very smooth.
- Pour into bowls and add a dollop of the sour cream to each, swirling it in.

50. No-lettuce leftovers salad

Ingredients

- 1 carrots spiralized
- 2 radishes thinly sliced
- 1/2 cup celery leaves
- 1/4 cup zucchini or other bits of vegetables
- Leftovers mustard dressing
- 1 tbsp mustard (prepared) any kind, in the bottom of the jar
- 3 tbsp olive oil (extra virgin)
- 1 tbsp apple cider vinegar

Instructions

- Spiralize a carrot or zucchini as the base of your salad. If you don't have a spiralizer, use a peeler like I do in the video to create carrot ribbons. Thinly slice any other vegetables you have, including the end pieces after spiralizing, the celery leaves, radishes, etc. Build your plate.

- If you have any odds and ends of fresh herbs, chop them and add them too!
- Add oil and vinegar to the mustard jar and shake well until emulsified. Drizzle over the salad and enjoy.

51.   Roasted carrot bisque

INGREDIENTS

- 2 pounds carrots peeled, cut into chunks
- 1 onions peeled, halved, then quartered (use white parts of one bunch of green onions for the MRP migraine diet)
- 2 cloves garlic peeled
- 1-1/2 tablespoons coconut oil melted, or extra virgin olive oil
- 1-1/2 tablespoons honey maple syrup for vegan version; omit for MRP and Whole30
- 4 cups chicken stock (low-sodium) or low-sodium vegetable broth
- 14 ounces coconut milk canned, full-fat
- 1-1/2 cups water (filtered or spring)
- 1 teaspoon sea salt omit for MRP or low-sodium diets
- 1/8 teaspoon black pepper

Instructions

- Preheat your oven to 425F/220C/gas mark 6.5.
- Place the carrots, onion, and garlic cloves on a large rimmed baking sheet and toss with the oil and sweetener to coat. Spread out the vegetables into a single layer.
- Roast for 20 minutes. Stir and spread the vegetables back into a single layer. Roast for 20 to 25 more minutes, or until soft and browned around the edges, but not burned.
- Transfer the roasted vegetables to your blender or food processor and add the broth. Blend for 2 to 3 minutes, or until relatively smooth. This may need to be done in two batches.
- Pour the carrot mixture into a large saucepan over medium-low heat. Stir in the coconut milk and desired amount of water to thin. Season with the salt and pepper to taste. Cook until heated through.
- Ladle into bowls. If desired, swirl with a little coconut cream or coconut milk and sprinkle with minced fresh parsley.
- Store leftovers in an airtight container in the refrigerator for up to 2 days.

52.   Watermelon salad with tofu

INGREDIENTS

- 2 pounds watermelon seedless
- 2 cucumbers large
- 4 ounces tofu firm, tofu feta, or regular feta
- 1 limes
- 1 tbsp olive oil (extra virgin) citrus-infused if possible
- 1 lime leaves optional
- 1 handful mint leaves (fresh) orange-mint or peppermint
- 1 tsp sea salt
- 1 pinch white pepper
- 1 handful Italian flat-leaf parsley (fresh)

Instructions

- Cut up the watermelon into small chunks.
- Peel the cucumbers and cut in half lengthwise. Scrape out the seeds with a grapefruit spoon. Cut into slices and add to the salad bowl with the watermelon.
- Juice the lime. Add the oil, salt, and white pepper to the lime juice and whisk. Pour over the contents of the bowl.
- Fold the Southeast Asian lime leaf in half, and cut away the hard vein running down the center.
- Finely chop the Southeast Asian lime leaf and the mint. Add to the bowl.
- Crumble the tofu feta. Add to the bowl. Toss. Add additional salt if needed after tasting. Top with a little bit of parsley if desired

53.   Curried greens

Ingredients

- 12-16 ounces kale also Swiss chard, beet, turnip, mustard, etc.
- 2 cloves garlic
- 1 tbsp olive oil (extra virgin) or coconut oil
- 3-4 tsp curry powder mild or medium
- 14 ounces coconut milk light or regular

INSTRUCTIONS

- Wash and dry the greens.
- Finely chop the greens (stems too!) by pulsing in the food processor, a handful at a time. You want them finely chopped but not puréed.
- Smash the garlic cloves, remove the papery husks, and finely mince.
- Minced Garlic for curried greens
- Heat the oil in a cast iron frying pan or non-stick sauté pan.
- Add the curry powder and garlic and cook for just a minute.
- Sauteeing the Curry powder and garlic for curried greens

- Add the greens and cook, stirring every few minutes, for about five minutes until they start to wilt.
- Add the coconut milk and stir, mixing thoroughly.
- Adding coconut milk to curried greens
- Bring to a boil, then turn down to simmer, cover, and cook for 30-60 minutes. Top with a sprinkle of red pepper flakes if desired (shown).

54. Paleo dirty rice

Ingredients

- 2 tbsp olive oil (extra virgin) or rendered high-quality bacon fat
- 1-1/2 cups celery diced, with leaves (about 4 stalks)
- 2 cloves garlic
- 2 bell peppers red, diced
- 16 ounces turkey chorizo Diestel Farms
- 3 cups cauliflower (riced)
- 16 ounces kale or Swiss chard, chopped
- 2 tbsp cilantro can sub fresh Italian flat-leaf parsley if you hate cilantro
- 1/2 cup chicken stock (low-sodium) (if dry)

Instructions

- Heat the oil in a large Dutch oven over medium heat until shimmering.
- Sauté the celery for five minutes until softening and golden. Add the garlic, bell peppers and cook for 1 minute.
- Add the turkey and cook, breaking up, for 5 minutes.
- Add the remaining ingredients and cook for 25 minutes until the flavors are melded.
- Serve at once. This freezes well and makes excellent lunches or dinners.

55.   Antipasto Skewers

Ingredients:

- Cherry tomatoes
- Mozzarella balls (bocconcini)
- Sliced salami or prosciutto
- Pitted olives (such as Kalamata or green)
- Basil leaves
- Balsamic glaze (optional)
- Wooden skewers

Instructions:

- Thread cherry tomatoes, mozzarella balls, sliced salami or prosciutto, pitted olives, and basil leaves onto wooden skewers in desired order.
- Arrange the skewers on a serving platter.

- Drizzle with balsamic glaze, if desired, before serving.

56.   Vegetable and Lentil Curry

Ingredients:

- 1 cup dried green or brown lentils, rinsed
- 2 cups low-sodium vegetable broth
- 1 tablespoon olive oil
- 1 onion, diced
- 2 cloves garlic, minced
- 1 tablespoon grated fresh ginger
- 2 carrots, diced
- 2 potatoes, diced
- 1 can (14 oz) diced tomatoes
- 1 can (14 oz) coconut milk
- 2 tablespoons curry powder
- 1 teaspoon ground cumin
- Salt and pepper to taste
- Cooked rice or naan bread, for serving

Instructions:

- In a large pot, heat olive oil over medium heat. Add diced onion, minced garlic, and grated ginger. Cook until fragrant, about 2 minutes.
- Add diced carrots and potatoes to the pot. Cook for another 5 minutes, stirring occasionally.
- Stir in curry powder and ground cumin, coating the vegetables evenly.

- Add rinsed lentils, vegetable broth, diced tomatoes (with their juices), and coconut milk to the pot. Stir to combine.
- Bring the mixture to a boil, then reduce heat to low and simmer for 20-25 minutes, or until lentils and vegetables are tender and the curry has thickened.
- Season with salt and pepper to taste.
- Serve the vegetable and lentil curry hot over cooked rice or with naan bread for a comforting and flavorful dinner.

57.   Coconut Rice Pudding

Ingredients:

- 1 cup cooked rice (such as jasmine or basmati)
- 1 can (14 oz) coconut milk
- 1/4 cup maple syrup or honey
- 1 teaspoon vanilla extract
- 1/4 teaspoon ground cinnamon
- Pinch of salt
- Toasted coconut flakes for garnish (optional)

Instructions:

- In a saucepan, combine cooked rice, coconut milk, maple syrup or honey, vanilla extract, ground cinnamon, and a pinch of salt.
- Bring the mixture to a simmer over medium heat, stirring occasionally.
- Reduce heat to low and simmer gently for 20-25 minutes, stirring occasionally, until the rice pudding thickens.

- Remove from heat and let cool slightly before serving.
- Serve warm or chilled, garnished with toasted coconut flakes if desired. Enjoy this creamy and comforting coconut rice pudding as a delightful dessert.

58.   Spinach and Mushroom Frittata

Ingredients:

- 6 eggs
- 1 cup fresh spinach, chopped
- 1/2 cup sliced mushrooms
- 1/4 cup diced onion
- 1/4 cup shredded cheese (such as cheddar or mozzarella)
- 1 tablespoon olive oil
- Salt and pepper to taste

Instructions:

- Preheat the oven to 350°F (175°C).
- In a mixing bowl, whisk together the eggs, salt, and pepper until well combined.
- Heat olive oil in an oven-safe skillet over medium heat. Add the diced onion and sliced mushrooms, and cook until softened.
- Add the chopped spinach to the skillet and cook until wilted.
- Pour the whisked eggs over the vegetables in the skillet. Allow the mixture to cook undisturbed for a few minutes until the edges start to set.

- Sprinkle the shredded cheese evenly over the top of the frittata.
- Transfer the skillet to the preheated oven and bake for 12-15 minutes, or until the eggs are fully set and the cheese is melted and bubbly.
- Remove from the oven, slice into wedges, and serve hot.

59.   Mediterranean Chickpea Salad

Ingredients:

- 1 can (15 oz) chickpeas, drained and rinsed
- 1 cucumber, diced
- 1 bell pepper, diced
- 1 cup cherry tomatoes, halved
- 1/4 cup red onion, thinly sliced
- 1/4 cup Kalamata olives, pitted and halved
- 2 tablespoons chopped fresh parsley
- 2 tablespoons extra virgin olive oil
- 1 tablespoon red wine vinegar
- 1 teaspoon dried oregano
- Salt and pepper to taste

Instructions:

- In a large mixing bowl, combine the chickpeas, diced cucumber, diced bell pepper, halved cherry tomatoes, sliced red onion, halved Kalamata olives, and chopped fresh parsley.

- In a small bowl, whisk together the extra virgin olive oil, red wine vinegar, dried oregano, salt, and pepper to make the dressing.
- Pour the dressing over the chickpea salad and toss until well coated.
- Refrigerate the salad for at least 30 minutes to allow the flavors to meld before serving.
- Serve chilled as a refreshing and satisfying lunch option.

60. Turkey and Vegetable Stir-Fry

Ingredients:

- 1 lb turkey breast, thinly sliced
- 2 cups mixed vegetables (such as broccoli florets, bell peppers, snap peas, carrots)
- 2 cloves garlic, minced
- 2 tablespoons low-sodium soy sauce
- 1 tablespoon hoisin sauce
- 1 tablespoon sesame oil
- Cooked rice or noodles, for serving
- Sesame seeds and chopped green onions for garnish (optional)

Instructions:

- Heat sesame oil in a large skillet or wok over medium-high heat.
- Add minced garlic to the skillet and cook until fragrant, about 30 seconds.

- Add thinly sliced turkey breast to the skillet and stir-fry until cooked through.
- Add mixed vegetables to the skillet and stir-fry until crisp-tender.
- In a small bowl, whisk together low-sodium soy sauce and hoisin sauce. Pour the sauce over the turkey and vegetables in the skillet.
- Cook for an additional 1-2 minutes, stirring constantly, until the sauce thickens and coats the turkey and vegetables.
- Serve the turkey and vegetable stir-fry hot over cooked rice or noodles.

61.   Berry Coconut Chia Seed Popsicles

Ingredients:

- 1 cup mixed berries (such as strawberries, blueberries, raspberries)
- 1 can (14 oz) coconut milk
- 2 tablespoons chia seeds
- 2 tablespoons honey or maple syrup
- Popsicle molds and sticks

Instructions:

- In a blender, puree the mixed berries until smooth.
- In a mixing bowl, combine the coconut milk, chia seeds, and honey or maple syrup. Stir until well combined.
- Pour the berry puree into the coconut milk mixture and stir gently to create a marbled effect.

- Pour the mixture into popsicle molds, filling each mold about three-quarters full.
- Insert popsicle sticks into the molds and freeze for at least 4 hours, or until the popsicles are firm.
- Once frozen, remove the popsicles from the molds and serve immediately.

62.   Blueberry Almond Overnight Oats

Ingredients:

- 1/2 cup rolled oats
- 1/2 cup low-tyramine milk alternative (such as almond milk or oat milk)
- 1/4 cup plain Greek yogurt (low-tyramine)
- 1/4 cup fresh blueberries
- 1 tablespoon almond butter
- 1 teaspoon honey or maple syrup
- 1/2 teaspoon vanilla extract

Instructions:

- In a mason jar or container, combine rolled oats, low-tyramine milk alternative, plain Greek yogurt, almond butter, honey or maple syrup, and vanilla extract.
- Stir in fresh blueberries.
- Cover the jar with a lid and refrigerate overnight, or for at least 4 hours.

63.   Tuna Salad Lettuce Wraps

Ingredients:

- 1 can (5 oz) tuna, drained
- 2 tablespoons Greek yogurt (low-tyramine)
- 1 tablespoon lemon juice
- 1/4 cup diced celery
- 1/4 cup diced red onion
- 1 tablespoon chopped fresh parsley
- Salt and pepper to taste
- Lettuce leaves (such as butter lettuce or romaine) for wrapping

Instructions:

- In a mixing bowl, combine drained tuna, Greek yogurt, lemon juice, diced celery, diced red onion, chopped fresh parsley, salt, and pepper.
- Stir until well combined and the tuna salad is evenly mixed.
- Spoon the tuna salad mixture onto lettuce leaves.
- Wrap the lettuce leaves around the tuna salad filling to create lettuce wraps.
- Serve immediately as a light and refreshing lunch option.

64.   Beef and bean soup

INGREDIENTS

- 1 pound dried beans SOAKED OVERNIGHT in filtered or spring water. I used a 10-bean blend. Use any of these for the migraine diet: chickpeas, white beans, kidney beans, split peas, black beans,
- 2 tbsp olive oil (extra virgin)
- 1 onions diced. Use a bunch of green onions for the migraine diet.
- 2 cloves garlic minced
- 2 carrots peeled and sliced into coins
- 2 potatoes new or Yukon gold (but any type will do), large dice
- 4 ounces beef (grass-fed) pork or lamb, cubed (can omit to make this vegan)
- 4 cups water (filtered or spring)
- 1/4 cup tomato paste or red pepper paste/puree
- 3 bay leaves
- 3 thyme (fresh) 2-3 sprigs
- 1 tbsp Italian seasoning salt-free OR Porcini Paradiso from Spice Tribe

INSTRUCTIONS

- Soak the dried beans overnight in plenty of water. If possible, use filtered or spring water for the best flavor. Rinse and drain.
- Heat the oil in the Instant Pot set to Saute (medium heat level). Saute the onion, garlic, and carrots for 5 minutes or until turning golden.
- Add the Italian seasoning and cook for 1 minute to release the oils.

- Add remaining ingredients and stir well, making sure the tomato paste is dissolved. Hit Cancel.
- Secure the lid, then set to Pressure Cook on high for 25 minutes. Use natural pressure release. After opening the lid, remove the 3 bay leaves and the thyme sprigs. Serve hot, garnished with more fresh thyme if desired.

65.   Salmon potato cakes

INGREDIENTS

- 6 ounces salmon canned, Alaskan pink, no salt added
- ounces potatoes grated (1 cup)
- 3 ounces carrots grated (1 small or 1/2 large)
- 2 ounces bell peppers red, about 1/4 pepper
- 1 eggs local, free-range (outdoors if possible)
- 4 tbsp flax seeds (ground)
- 2 tbsp half and half organic
- 1 tsp Old Bay seasoning homemade for low-sodium diet
- 1 tsp garlic powder
- 1/2 tsp dill weed (dried)
- 1/4 tsp black pepper

INSTRUCTIONS

- Drain the salmon and flake it into a large mixing bowl.
- Measure and add the potatoes.

- Put the carrot in the food processor and pulse until roughly chopped. Add the red bell pepper and pulse until both are fairly finely chopped, but do not overwork it.
- Add the carrot, bell pepper, and remaining ingredients to the bowl and mix with a spatula until evenly distributed.
- Let sit 20 minutes.
- Preheat the Foreman grill, grill pan, or non-stick frying pan.
- Use the spatula to smoosh everything together, so that the potato starch and the flax seeds make it very sticky.
- Use a measuring cup, egg ring, or ice cream scoop to portion out the patties evenly.
- Cook for five minutes per side.